Fit for Adventure

A Comprehensive Guide for Fitness Enthusiasts and Nutrition Geeks

Table of Contents

Chapter 1. Introduction

Welcome aboard fellow adventurers! Get ready for an exciting journey into exceptional fitness and nutrition insights from our special report, "Fit for Adventure: A Comprehensive Guide for Fitness Enthusiasts and Nutrition Geeks." Dive deep into riveting narratives about physical prowess, unfastened from the shackles of complicated terminology. We bring together exclusive interviews from industry professionals, holistic advice from expert nutritionists, and landmark studies, all curated to empower you on your health journey. This comprehensive guide is designed to inspire, inform and most importantly, instigate change that leads to an upgraded, adventure-ready you! Trust us when we say that this is not just a purchase, it's an investment you make for your body and mind.

Chapter 2. Footing the Foundations: Building the Fitness Mindset

Before you can embark on a physical journey of transformation and adventure, it's imperative to kick off the empowerment with a mental makeover. The mindset with which you approach fitness is fundamental to the success of your journey, shaping your commitment, endurance, and ultimately, your results. This section will delve into the nuanced equation of creating a sustainable, success-fostering fitness mindset.

2.1. Fundamentals of a Fitness Mindset

Adopting a fitness mindset involves much more than scheduling workout sessions and pushing your body to its limits. It starts firmly in your mind, with your thoughts, attitudes, and perceptions influencing your ultimate success more than any set of dumbbells or fancy fitness equipment ever could.

1. Principle of Persistence: Consistency is the key that turns a fitness hopeful into a fitness achiever. Understanding it early on saves you from the damning loop of sporadic bursts of activity followed by long spells of inactivity. Remember, the path to physical prowess isn't conquered in a day.

2. Embracing Discomfort: Physical training isn't easy, and it isn't meant to be. By acknowledging and witnessing the discomfort as a sign of growth, it becomes a stepping stone rather than an insurmountable obstacle.

3. Positive Reinforcement: Success in fitness requires recognizing

and celebrating small victories. Completing a challenging workout, adding a few more pounds to your lift, even sticking to your planned schedule – these milestones deserve recognition and will fuel your motivation.

2.2. Redefining Goals: The SMART Way

Traditional goal-setting methods often fail to deliver tangible results. However, when you break down your fitness aspirations using the SMART methodology, you amp up your chance at success. SMART stands for Specific, Measurable, Achievable, Relevant, and Time-bound.

1. Specific: Having a clear and specific goal in mind helps focus your efforts. Instead of aiming for 'getting fit', target more explicit objectives, say, 'being able to run 5 miles without stopping.'

2. Measurable: Trackable progress allows you to see how far you've come and how much remains to be accomplished. This could be minutes shaved off your run, extra reps added to your weights routine, or pounds/inches lost/gained.

3. Achievable: Set goals that stretch you but are still within your reach. Aiming too high can lead to frustration and early burnout.

4. Relevant: Your fitness goals must be in alignment with your larger life goals. Ensuring relevance safeguards against fitness becoming a chore.

5. Time-bound: Deadlines spur action. Set a completion date for your goals without falling into the trap of setting unrealistic timeframes.

2.3. Mind Over Muscle: The Power of Visualization

Visualization is an often-underlooked facet of the fitness journey. It involves using your imagination to create mental images of what you want to achieve. Visualizing your success, be it finishing a marathon in under four hours or scaling the steepest climbing wall, creates a neural pathway that helps your body understand and adapt to what it needs to do to realize this vision. This mental rehearsal can also boost motivation and commitment.

2.4. Arms and Armor: Tools for a Resilient Mindset

While setting goals and visualizing success are critical steps in crafting your fitness mindset, it's essential to have a contingency plan for when the going gets tough. Here are some tools to fortify your mental resilience:

1. Meditation: This age-old practice has been scientifically proven to reduce stress and anxiety, improve focus, and promote a sense of calm – all beneficial to maintaining your fitness commitment.

2. Affirmations: Positive self-talk helps combat self-doubt and negativity. Creating an affirmation unique to your fitness journey can perk up motivation, self-belief, and strength of mind.

3. Mindful Movement: Engaging in activities like yoga, Tai Chi or Pilates can enhance body awareness, instill discipline and deepen the psychological connection to your fitness journey.

2.5. The Sustenance Spectrum: Mental Diet for a Fitness Mindset

Just as your body needs proper nutrition to perform optimally, your mind also needs a wholesome mental diet. Consuming positive, elevating content while distancing yourself from negativity, time-wasting distractions, and defeatist attitudes nourishes your fitness mindset and keeps it in peak condition.

2.6. The Ripple Effect: The Wider Impact of a Fitness Mindset

A fitness mindset doesn't just elevate your workout regimen; it has implications far beyond the gym walls. Embracing persistence, resilience, goal orientation, and a positive outlook seeps into every other aspect of your life. It enhances self-esteem, resilience, and overall well-being.

Armed with these insights, it's time to fire up your mental engines, craft your fitness mindset, and set forth on the path of health-filled adventure. Remember, every step, every rep, and every morsel of nutritious food is a victorious battle in the greater war for outstanding fitness and exceptional health. Forge ahead with persistence and positivity; your fit, adventure-ready self is waiting!

Chapter 3. Choosing your Path: Identifying Your Activity Profile

Just as you would plan a route before embarking on a physical journey, the path to fitness also begins with determined direction, an understanding of your strengths, and an accommodation for your weaknesses. This chapter is dedicated to assisting you in identifying your activity profile, a concrete platform from which you can leap into a new world of fitness and nutrition. By understanding your current activity levels, fitness strengths, limitations, and preferences, you can devise a personalized exercise plan that not only benefits your body but also harmonizes with your life.

3.1. Understanding Your Baseline

The first step towards establishing your activity profile is understanding your current physical activity level or baseline. Assess the intensity, duration, and types of physical activities that you perform likely daily.

The key to determining your activity baseline is honesty. It's easy to overestimate the time spent being physically active and underestimate the time spent being sedentary. To avoid this, try recording your activities for a week. This could include your time spent walking, running, household chores, climbing stairs, gardening, or any other form of physical exertion. Equally important is to notice passive activities like watching TV or working at a desk.

Now that you have a clear vision of your current activity levels, categorize them into three basic activity categories; sedentary, moderate, and vigorous.

- **Sedentary** activities include sitting or reclining (watching TV, reading, desk work, etc.)

- **Moderate** activities require moderate physical effort and cause small increases in breathing or heart rate (e.g. brisk walking, sweeping the floor, cycling for pleasure, etc.)

- **Vigorous** activities demand hard physical effort and result in substantial increases in breathing or heart rate (like running, swimming laps, aerobics, etc.)

Assign each activity from your record to one of these categories to baseline your physical activity profile.

3.2. Assessing Fitness Capabilities

Understanding your fitness capabilities can provide a useful guide for formulating a practical exercise schedule and monitoring progress. There are five primary components to general fitness, each requiring different types of exercises to improve. These are cardiovascular endurance, muscular strength, muscular endurance, flexibility, and body composition.

You can perform simple self-tests to assess each of these components, like measuring how long you can run without stopping for cardiovascular endurance, or how many push-ups you can do without rest for muscular strength.

Testing these aspects can be insightful in two primary ways. Firstly, knowing your fitness capabilities will make it easier to recognize your strengths that can be capitalized upon, and weaknesses that need more attention. Secondly, it provides a starting point from which you can track your improvements over time.

3.3. Identifying Your Preferences

Now that you're more familiar with your baseline and your fitness abilities, the next element to consider are your preferences. No matter how beneficial an exercise is, if you dread doing it each day, the chances of sticking with it are slim. Instead, identifying physical activities that you genuinely enjoy can make your journey to fitness more enjoyable and sustainable in the long run.

In addition to personal likes and dislikes, lifestyle factors such as available time, work schedule, family commitments, and access to facilities or equipment should be considered while developing your activity profile.

3.4. Developing a Personalized Activity Profile

Drawing from your understanding of your activity baseline, fitness capabilities, and preferences, you can now develop an enhanced activity profile. This profile forms the basis of your individualized exercise plan.

Try to build a plan that varies in types of activities. Aim for a balance between cardiovascular endurance exercises (like running, swimming, biking), strength training (like weight lifting, resistance band exercises), and flexibility exercises (like yoga, stretching). This ensures a comprehensive approach.

Additionally, align this plan with your preferences. Including activities you enjoy guarantees that your exercise regimen is not just efficient, but also enjoyable.

3.5. Embarking on Your Journey

Identifying your activity profile is an empowering first step, but your journey has only just begun. The persistence to stay committed to your plan and the flexibility to adjust your activities based on progress, personal experiences, and new preferences is crucial.

Remember that fitness is not a race but a lifelong process. Be patient with yourself and celebrate every little progress. After all, every push-up, every lap, every skipped dessert is a step towards an adventure-ready you, fashioned by this comprehensive guide.

The highest peaks are ascended not in leaps, but in small determined steps. Embark on your fitness adventure your way, at your pace, and enjoy the journey as much as the destination. The path to being 'Fit for Adventure' waits for you!

Chapter 4. Mapping the Compass: Understanding Basic Anatomy

Human beings are masterpieces of design. We are an amalgamation of complex organs and systems that synergistically work together, enabling us to perform both mundane and heroic feats. Today, in our quest for better fitness and nutrition, we delve into the intricacies of our basic anatomy. Buckle up as we evaluate each component's unique attributes, functions, and the vital role they play in maintaining our health and fitness.

4.1. The Muscular System

All actions, from lifting weights to running a marathon, are made possible through the harmonious function of our muscles. More than 600 muscles are in our body, and they comprise nearly half of a person's total body weight, making an understanding of the muscular system integral to fitness.

Muscles are classified into three types:

1. Skeletal muscles: Attached to bones, they are responsible for all voluntary movements like walking or grabbing a glass of water.

2. Smooth muscles: Found in organs and structures like the esophagus, stomach, intestines, bronchi, uterus, urethra, blood vessels, and the skin, they control involuntary movements.

3. Cardiac muscles: Found exclusively in the heart, they are responsible for pumping blood throughout the body.

Each muscle is composed of muscle fibers (muscle cells), where the interaction of proteins myosin and actin results in contraction, causing movement. This understanding is pivotal when aiming for muscle hypertrophy (growth) or increasing strength and endurance in a fitness regimen.

4.2. The Skeletal System

No discussion about muscles can be complete without referencing the skeletal structure to which muscles attach and leverage to cause movement. The human body has 206 bones that not only act as a frame giving us shape, but also provide protection to vital organs, produce blood cells, and store vital minerals.

The skeletal system is classified into two, namely:

1. Axial Skeleton: It consists of the skull, vertebral column, chest, and rib cage, crucial for protecting vital organs.

2. Appendicular Skeleton: It includes the pectoral and pelvic girdles along with the limbs, essential for locomotion.

To ensure optimal fitness, maintaining bone health is paramount. Weight-bearing exercises, such as running, hiking, weightlifting, help increase bone density, providing resistance against fractures and osteoporosis.

4.3. The Cardiovascular System

The cardiovascular system is an intricate network comprising the heart, blood, and blood vessels, responsible for transporting oxygen, nutrients, hormones, and cellular waste products throughout the body.

The heart, a four-chambered muscular organ, plays a crucial role in pumping oxygen and nutrient-rich blood to all body parts, thereby making it pivotal in stamina-building exercises and cardiovascular fitness.

The system's efficacy can be enhanced by aerobic exercises like cycling, swimming, and running, which elevate heart rate and maximize nutrient and oxygen transportation.

4.4. The Digestive System

The saying "we are what we eat" rings especially true when discussing the digestive system, consisting of the gastrointestinal tract, liver, pancreas, and gallbladder. This system breaks down food into nutrients, which are absorbed to provide energy, growth, and cell repair.

For fitness enthusiasts, it's vital to consume nutrient-dense foods. Proteins aid in muscle recovery and growth, carbohydrates provide energy, and fats help with hormone production and nutrient absorption. Additionally, vigor in maintaining gut health can enhance nutrient absorption and foster overall well-being.

4.5. The Respiratory System

For any fitness endeavor, the respiratory system is vital. It involves the intake of oxygen and expulsion of carbon dioxide through a system that includes the nose, throat (pharynx and larynx), windpipe, and lungs. Regular cardiovascular and deep breathing exercises can heighten lung capacity and efficiency, enhancing overall physical performance.

In recognition of the connection between fitness and basic anatomy, one can pursue and attain desired health goals. Understand that exercises and nutrition affect not only our shape and size but, more importantly, our internal systems. By knowing and respecting our anatomy, we can optimally utilize our bodies to explore the endless realms of physical prowess.

Chapter 5. The Adventurer's Arsenal: Essential Fitness Equipment

Fitness and wellness aren't just about the time spent sweating in the gym. For sure, it is about that, but it also involves the tools and equipment we leverage in achieving our fitness dreams. In this comprehensive guide, we wheel through an investing in the right kind of training gear to satisfy your inner adventurer's appetite for fitness.

5.1. Choosing the Right Equipment

Embarking on a fitness journey isn't about owning the most expensive equipment but about understanding your needs and personal goals. Not all fitness tools are created equal; what works for your friends might not necessarily suit you. Consider your targeted areas, strength and flexibility level, and more importantly, your comfort. High-quality equipment should be easy to operate, adjustable, and have reliable safety features and long-term durability.

5.2. Cardio Equipment

Cardiovascular exercise is one of the fundamental aspects of any fitness regimen, boosting heart health and aiding in weight loss by increasing your metabolic rate.

Treadmills, stationary bikes, elliptical trainers, stair climbers, and rowing machines are among the common forms of cardio equipment that you can consider. These machines have adjustable resistances allowing for a range of workouts - from low impact to high intensity -

catering to all fitness levels.

5.3. Strength Equipment

Strength training, which fosters muscle growth, enhances bone density, and revs up your metabolism, is vital for maintaining overall body health.

Free weights like dumbbells, barbells, kettlebells are versatile and challenging, fostering strength, balance, and coordination. If you're new to weightlifting, adjustable dumbbells are a great pick—they offer multiple weight options in a single compact tool.

Weight machines, though less versatile, promote correct form and target specific muscle groups precisely, making them a favorite for beginners and rehabilitation.

Resistance bands are portable, affordable, and can effectively substitute their heavier counterparts for strength workouts.

5.4. Flexibility and Balance Equipment

Flexibility and balance training often get less attention, yet they are essential for preventing injuries and enhancing athletic performance.

Yoga mats provide a non-slip surface, essential for numerous stretching exercises, yoga or pilates.

Foam rollers serve as a useful accessory for self-myofascial release, helping to alleviate muscle stiffness and enhance muscle recovery.

Stability balls engage your core and improve balance while adding an extra challenge to your workout routine.

5.5. Home Gym Essentials

Building a home gym can be an excellent investment for those for whom travel or time constraints make hitting a public gym challenging.

The essentials for a home gym would include a yoga mat, a set of dumbbells, resistance bands, a stability ball, and a foam roller. Consider cardio machines if space and budget allow.

5.6. Outdoor Equipment

For those who prefer the great outdoors to a confined gym, there are several options.

Skipping ropes provide a quick and efficient cardio workout. Portable resistance bands can help you strengthen and tone wherever you are. Suspension trainers, which utilize body weight, can be attached to any secured anchor—like a tree or a door—and provide a full-body workout.

5.7. Technology and Fitness

No fitness arsenal would be complete without mentioning the tech tools that have burgeoned in the wellness space. Fitness trackers provide insightful data about heart rate, sleep patterns, step count, and calories burned, helping you stay informed and motivated. Plus, downloading fitness apps can provide structured workout plans, nutrition tips, and virtual community support right at your fingertips.

5.8. Maintaining Your Equipment

Investing in fitness equipment is just the beginning. Regular maintenance such as cleaning, inspection for wear and tear, and proper storage can go a long way in maintaining its utility and prolonging its lifetime.

Without a doubt, the right equipment can be a game-changer in your fitness journey, bringing variety, providing grip, and adding intensity. Taking the time to understand, choose wisely, and make full use of your fitness arsenal will fuel you on your mission to stay fit and ready for adventures.

Chapter 6. Climbing the Peak: Establishing Workout Routines

Before starting a journey, one needs to prepare diligently. As with any expedition, laying the groundwork for a solid fitness routine is essential. In this chapter, we will walk hand in hand with you through this process. Weaving together expert advice, scientific research, and first-hand testimonies, we aim to orient you through every nook and cranny of establishing an effective and enjoyable workout routine.

6.1. Creating a Fitness Vision

First, start by envisioning your peak. Your fitness goals are both your destination and your motivation. These objectives may vary vastly from person to person, influenced by factors such as your current fitness level, health condition, past experiences, or even long-harbored aspirations. However, make no mistake; setting attainable, measurable, realistic, and timed goals is of paramount importance.

Begin by asking the right questions. Why do you wish to workout? Is it to shed extra pounds? To pump up your strength and endurance levels for an upcoming marathon? Or perhaps to simply maintain a healthy lifestyle? Reflect on your answers and write them down. This will serve as a clear roadmap and tangible motivation for your fitness quest.

6.2. Starting Slow: The Importance of Building a Foundation

Once your goals are in sight, take it slowly. Starting on a high intensity or complicated workout routine may cause more harm than good. It's essential to meet yourself where you are, and to begin by slowly building strength and endurance. Incorporating low-intensity activities like walking, light jogging or strength exercises using your body weight may seem less flashy, yet is sure to yield incremental and sustainable results.

By building a strong fitness foundation, you not only prepare your body for more rigorous workouts down the line, you also enjoy the journey itself. Moreover, reducing the risk of injury and burnout is a critical aspect of maintaining long-term physical activity.

6.3. Enlisting Expert Guidance

Calling in the professionals is never a bad idea when it comes to getting fit. Personal trainers, physiotherapists, and even experienced friends can provide invaluable guidance regarding form, technique, frequency, and progress tracking. They can also give you effective tips on how to avoid common pitfalls and how to handle injury if it happens.

Keep in mind that personalised professional advice is no luxury, but an investment in your health. It ensures your efforts yield optimal results, and can help prevent demotivating setbacks due to injury or inefficient technique.

6.4. Creating a Customized Workout Routine

Now that you have goal clarity and foundational strength, and possibly some professional guidance, it's time to create the routine itself. Your workout routine should be tailored to suit your unique needs and circumstances. These could include preferred workout days and times, available equipment, workout duration, and even the type of exercises you find enjoyable.

Start with a mix of cardiovascular exercises and strength training, spreading them throughout your week in a balanced manner. Consistency is key, so ensure you have enough recovery time to avoid fatigue. Consider using online tools, fitness apps, or a simple notebook to plan and record your workouts.

Documenting fitness parameters like the weights, repetitions, and duration of each session is a worthwhile strategy for achieving progress. Pay attention to the subtle ways your body communicates its progress or distress, and adjust your routines proactively borrowing keen insights from your own data.

6.5. Nutrition: The Fuel for Your Journey

Let's not forget about the power of nutrition as a catalyst to power your workouts. Consuming a balanced diet packed with protein, complex carbohydrates, fruits and vegetables will not only support your body during grueling workout sessions, but enhance recovery and muscle growth post-workout.

Working with a dietitian or a nutritionist can provide professional advice on dietary adjustments tailored to your activity level, body composition, and fitness goals. Whether you're aiming for fat loss, muscle gain, or enhanced sports performance, having nutrition as a core element in your fitness plan will prove to be indispensable.

Chapter 7. Maintaining Flexibility, Rest & Recovery

Lastly, it's important to respect your body's need for rest and recovery. Adequate sleep, scheduled rest days, and recuperation practices like stretching, yoga, massage, or foam rolling, should be integral components of your program.

Remarkably, fitness is not just about being active, but also about taking care and listening to your body. The pursuit of strenuous exercise must always be balanced with honoring the body's need for calm, restoration, and rejuvenation.

In conclusion, embarking on the journey to fitness is like climbing a peak. It's not always easy, and requires planning, preparation and most importantly, consistency. It can sometimes be challenging, but the progress made more than makes up for the effort. Reaching the peak will not only be rewarding in itself, but the journey there will equip you with valuable insights about yourself, giving you a greater appreciation for your body's capabilities and endurance. Prepare well, start slow, enlist expert advice, customize to your needs, balance nutrition, and always remember to rest and recover. This is your journey, own it, and make it memorable. Happy climbing!

Chapter 8. The Tastemakers' Galley: Crafting the Ideal Nutrient-Packed Diet

Every fitness journey begins not with the first step on a treadmill or the first lift of a weight, but with the first bite of a healthy, balanced meal. Nutrition, the foundational cornerstone of any wellness program, plays a pivotal role in the achievement of your fitness goals. Whether you aim for weight loss, muscle gain, or simply maintaining a healthy lifestyle, understanding the complexities of nutrition can steer you towards success. This chapter will guide you to craft your nutrient-packed diet, helping you underpin your daily dietary needs.

8.1. The Keystone of Nutrition: Macros and Micronutrients

The cornerstone of nutrition rests upon two building blocks—macronutrients and micronutrients. Understanding these cornerstones may seem intimidating at first, but uncovering their essence can pave the way to profound insights.

Macronutrients comprise proteins, carbohydrates, and fats—elements required by our bodies in large quantities. Each plays a unique role.

1. Proteins: Essential for building and repairing tissues, proteins act as the building blocks of muscles, skin, enzymes, and hormones.

2. Carbohydrates: This is our body's preferred source of energy, used to fuel our daily movements and brain activities.

3. Fats: Contrary to popular belief, "good" fats provide energy,

support cell growth, protect organs, and even help absorb specific nutrients.

In addition to macronutrients, nutritionists emphasize the crucial role of micronutrients in a balanced diet. These include vitamins and minerals required in smaller quantities, yet they are vital for maintaining optimal health.

8.2. Crafting Your Macronutrient Strategy

Constructing your macronutrient strategy demands more than food intake quantification. It is about identifying your body's needs and tailoring your diet accordingly.

Here is a simple step-by-step guide:

1. Define Your 'Caloric Budget': Based on your fitness goals, calculate your Total Daily Energy Expenditure (TDEE). This is the total amount of calories your body requires to perform daily functions. It incorporates Basal Metabolic Rate (BMR), Physical Activity Level (PAL), and Thermic Effect of Food (TEF).

2. Adjust Your Caloric Intake: For weight loss, deduct 20-25% from your TDEE. For muscle gain, add 10-15% to your TDEE. For maintaining weight, stick to your calculated TDEE.

3. Determine Macronutrient Ratio: While there's no one-size-fits-all approach, a typical macro breakdown is 40% carbohydrates, 30% protein, and 30% fat. Specific fitness goals may prompt adjustments to these average ratios.

4. Customize Your Meal Plan: Now, divide your nutrient intake across meals, taking into account your unique preferences like meal frequency and timing constraints. You may benefit from specific dietary patterns like Paleo, Vegan, or Mediterranean, provided they align with your individual needs.

8.3. Enhancing Diet with Micronutrients

While macronutrients hold the spotlight, micronutrients deserve recognition. To fuel our bodies with the necessary vitamins and minerals, focus on consuming a varied, nutrient-dense diet. Here are key micronutrients for optimal health:

1. Vitamins: Consist of vitamins A, B, C, D, E, and K. They maintain the health of various body functions like the immune system, organs, skin, and bones.

2. Minerals: Important minerals include calcium, potassium, magnesium, iron, and zinc. These contribute to nerve function, bone health, muscle contraction, and fluid balance.

8.4. Nutritional Strategies for Different Fitness Goals

Different fitness objectives require varied nutritional approaches. Here's a brief overview:

1. Weight Loss: Incorporate a calorie deficit along with nutrient-dense foods. Lean protein helps preserve muscle mass. Fiber-rich vegetables improve satiety.

2. Muscle Gain: A slight caloric surplus is needed, with a focus on lean proteins to support muscle synthesis. Carbohydrates are necessary post-workout.

3. Performance Enhancement: Training athletes need higher carbohydrate intake for sustained energy. Adequate protein aids recovery and helps repair and build muscle.

4. Health Maintenance: A balanced diet rich in micronutrients with an emphasis on fruits, vegetables, lean proteins, whole grains,

and healthy fats supports overall wellness.

Crafting your diet, while it may seem strenuous, can profoundly impact your fitness journey. The importance of a nutritionally balanced diet cannot be understated. As the ancient physician Hippocrates stated, "Let food be thy medicine and medicine be thy food."

Chapter 9. Sustenance on the Road: Supplementing Your Journey

As the rhythm of your steps aligns with the cadence of your heartbeat, the path ahead becomes clearer. Those miles you've covered, the hills you've conquered, all that effort matters, but so does what fuels that effort. Yes, we're talking about nutrition - your primary fuel.

Fueling your body correctly not only optimizes your physical performance but also ensures the maintenance and recovery of your muscles. So, without any further ado, let's embark on a journey to explore the science and practicalities of sustenance on the road.

9.1. The Irrefutable Importance of Nutrition

Unbeatable physical prowess is indisputably the dream of every adventure enthusiast. To achieve this, nutrition plays a pivotal role. It provides us with the energy to power through our workouts, aids in muscle recovery, and helps maintain overall bodily functions. Essentially, think of nutrition as the fuel your sports car runs on. If you fill it with the wrong kind or quantity, the performance will dip significantly.

Scientific studies have consistently shown that proper nutrition has several benefits:

- Supports energy production and muscle function during workouts.
- Fuels the recovery process post-adventure or exercise.

- Boosts the immune system by providing necessary vitamins and minerals.

- Contributes to the prevention and management of chronic diseases like obesity, diabetes, and heart diseases.

Thus, it's clear that proper nutrition is an absolute non-negotiable for any fitness enthusiast.

9.2. Nourishing the Macro Way

As crucial as nutrition is, understanding it may seem like trying to decipher hieroglyphs. Fear not, for we're here to simplify it. First off, let's divide our food into three main categories: carbohydrates (carbs), proteins, and fats.

Carbohydrates are your primary source of energy. They break down into glucose, which fuels your muscles and your brain.

Proteins, on the other hand, are paramount for muscle recovery and growth. Every time you work out or go on an adventurous trek, your muscle tissues undergo microscopic wear and tear. Protein helps repair those tissues, enabling muscle growth and strength.

Finally, fats are essential for numerous functions, including absorbing vitamins, insulating and protecting vital organs, and acting as secondary energy sources when carbohydrate stores deplete.

For an active person, a balanced diet ideally consists of around 45-65% carbs, 10-35% protein, and 20-35% fats.

9.3. On-the-Go: Nutritious Meals and Snacks

When you're on the road, preparing balanced meals might not always be an option. This is where planning and packing the right kinds of meals and snacks become crucial. Consider foods that are portable, non-perishable, and nutrition-dense.

For proteins, think about packing a couple of hard-boiled eggs, roasted chickpeas, or a jar of peanut butter. Fruits like bananas and oranges make for good carb sources that are easy to pack. Nuts and seeds can provide the necessary fats along with an energy boost.

Hydration is just as important. Always carry a water bottle. For extra-long activities, consider sports drinks to replenish lost electrolytes.

9.4. Supplements: A Boon to Your Journey

In a world that demands constant motion and progress, supplements can provide that extra edge needed to meet nutritional requirements.

However, supplements are not meant to replace a balanced diet but rather to support it. Consumption should be specific, taking into account your personal dietary needs, fitness goals, and any nutrient gaps in your diet.

Here are a few supplements that could prove advantageous:

- Whey Protein: For quicker recovery and muscle growth.
- Creatine: For boosting strength and muscle mass.
- Vitamin D: For bone health and immune system support.
- Electrolyte Supplements: For maintaining hydration and proper muscle function.

Before starting any supplement regimen, it's critical to consult a healthcare professional. Not all bodies function similarly; your healthcare provider can guide you based on your specific needs, medical history, and activity levels.

9.5. Small Changes, Big Excursions

Remember, the aim is not to overhaul your eating habits overnight. Instead, make small, steady changes by introducing new foods to your diet gradually. Monitor how your body reacts to these additions and adjust accordingly. Most importantly, keep your meals colorful, tasty, and enjoyable.

Remember that the path to fitness is not a sprint; it's a long, beautiful hike. May every step you make be stirred by a heart that's not just fit but also well-nourished. Enjoy the journey – it's worth every single step!

Chapter 10. Conserving Resources: The Importance of Rest and Recovery

In the wide-ranging universe of health and fitness, the accent on exercise and nutrition is prominent. However, one less-glamorous yet equally essential component is often overlooked: 'rest and recovery'. This chapter unravels the critical influence of rest and recovery on your transformative health journey, equipped with scientific data, expert advice, and fascinating anecdotes.

10.1. The Science of Rest and Recovery

Understanding the science of rest and recovery begins with appreciating its dual-purpose: repair and reinforcement. Whenever we exercise, our body breaks down muscle tissues, leading to minute tears. As alarming as that may sound, it's part of the process. It's during rest that the body repairs these tissues, fortifying them in the process, promoting muscle growth and strength.

Your body's endocrine and immune systems play pivotal roles during this recovery period. Hormones like insulin, testosterone, and human growth hormone work align to reestablish energy stores and repair tissue damage. The immune system, on the other hand, helps manage the inflammation induced by exercise.

Understanding this intricate biological synchrony underscores the imperativeness of a balanced rest and recovery plan, without which you risk counterproductive overtraining, fatigue, and potential injuries.

10.2. Pillars of Recovery

The practice of recovery is more nuanced than merely halting physical activity. It's a composition of various contributory components.

10.3. The Dangers of Neglecting Recovery

Mindful practices: Stress management techniques like meditation and mindfulness help in mental recovery, facilitating better sleep and overall well-being.

When recovery is compromised, acute effects like fatigue or muscle pain can translate into long-term implications such as chronic injuries, hormone imbalance, and an increased risk of illnesses due to a weakened immune system. These consequences hinder progress, proving detrimental to achieving your fitness goals.

More critically, overtraining without sufficient recovery can spur mental health issues, such as increased susceptibility to mood swings, anxiety, and depression. The assurance here is not to instill fear, but to underline the importance of an optimized recovery process.

10.4. Personalizing Your Recovery

Just as every individual's fitness and nutritional requirements vary, so do their recovery needs. Factors influencing this include the type of physical activity one partakes in, their age, fitness level, lifestyle factors etc. It's certainly beneficial to seek personalized guidance from professionals to curate a recovery plan best suited to your needs.

10.5. Recovery Indicators

Finally, it's practical to monitor recovery to adjust interventions as necessary. Here are some common indicators:

Listen to Your Body: Finally, cultivate an in tune relationship with your body. It will invariably reveal when it's time to rest and recover.

As we draw the curtains on this chapter, let's recapture the central takeaways: Rest and recovery hold a station of paramount importance on your fitness journey. Embrace this element of your regimen as passionately as you do your workouts and nutrition, and embark on your tailored journey towards 'Fit for Adventure'. With proper rest and recovery, you can conserve your resources, enhance your physical prowess, and foster a healthier mind-body confluence, truly being fit for any and every venture your adventurous spirit yearns for. You're not just buying into a health journey; you're investing in a life enriched with vitality, vigour and endless potential for astounding adventures.

Chapter 11. Battlefield Strategies: Injury Prevention and Management

Understanding how to prevent and manage injuries is a crucial component of any fitness journey. From minor sprains to serious conditions, how we tend to our bodies during these times of duress can make the difference between a quick recovery and a breakthrough to further injury.

11.1. The Anatomy of Injury

Before delving into injury management, it's vital to explore why injuries happen. They're typically due to imbalances in the body, overuse of certain muscle groups, or incorrect body mechanics during exercise. This means that knowing your body and respecting its limits plays a crucial role in injury prevention.

11.2. Weapons for War: A Healthy Arsenal

This sub-chapter will take you through steps towards better injury prevention. A key defense mechanism against injuries is a well-rounded fitness routine consisting of cardiovascular, strength, and flexibility exercises.

Cardiovascular exercises boost heart health, providing muscles with ample oxygen during exercise. This reduces fatigue and prevents injuries related to muscle strains.

Strength training, in turn, boosts muscle mass and joint stability. This helps in two ways: first, it provides a larger base of support reducing the chance of imbalance, and second, it reduces the likelihood of muscle strains and joint injuries.

Flexibility exercises boost your movement range and may help to prevent injuries typically associated with sudden movements or strains.

A balanced diet filled with lean proteins, quality carbs, healthy fats, and a variety of fruits and vegetables further aids injury prevention. Nutrients such as Vitamin D, Calcium, and Omega-3 fatty acids are especially important for bone health and inflammation reduction.

===Mobilize and Diversify: The Key Tactics

It is not just what you do but how you do it that matters. Proper form and technique trump mindless repetitions. Having more variety in your workouts also allows different muscle groups to rest, reducing injury risks attached to overuse.

11.3. Critical Care: Injury Management

What if an injury occurs despite your best efforts for prevention? In such cases, immediate first aid using the RICE (Rest, Ice, Compress, and Elevation) protocol may prevent further injury and inflammation. Rest allows the injured site to heal, ice reduces swelling, compression aids in reducing inflammation, and elevation helps in draining excessive fluids.

11.4. Call For Reinforcements: Seeking Medical Help

If the injury is severe or if symptoms persist, getting professional medical help is critical. A healthcare professional can provide a proper diagnosis and treatment plan. Follow-up care, like participating in physical rehabilitation or physiotherapy, may also be suggested to restore normal movement and function.

11.5. Battle Scars: Recurrent Injuries

Recurrent injuries usually signal an unresolved issue or a rushed return to intense physical activity. Here, the aid of a fitness specialist may be invaluable. They can help identify and correct faulty movement patterns while providing a safe, gradual return-to-play plan.

11.6. The Champion's Rest: Importance of Recovery

Rest and recovery are underestimated components of a fitness journey. The body repairs itself during periods of rest. So not taking enough time off can lead to overuse injuries. Consider employing strategies like active recovery, proper sleep, and hydration to aid your regeneration processes.

11.7. Nourish to Flourish: Post-Injury Nutrition

Floating on the raft of recovery also demands attention towards a nutritious diet, with key focus on protein for muscle repair, Vitamin C for collagen production, and antioxidants for inflammation reduction.

Injury prevention, immediate care, professional help, recovery, and nutrition - your blueprint for navigating fitness injuries is now complete. With this knowledge, you'll be more than prepared to journey through the frontlines of physical fitness without undue harm. Remember, an obstacle is often a stepping stone. Stay strong, stay safe, and keep adventuring!

Chapter 12. Ascend Beyond: Advanced Techniques for the Experienced Fitness Enthusiast

You've honed your fitness regimen to a fine edge. Your body is steady as a rock, flexible as a tendril, and you have strength that is impressive. But isn't there more to fitness? Yes, there is! Advanced techniques require commitment, understanding, and precision. They can elevate your fitness levels beyond your regular routine and create a significant difference in your overall wellbeing. They could range from enhancing your workout protocols to employing meditation – every addition aims to drive you past your limits and toward exceptional health and wellness.

Let's explore these techniques and how to incorporate them into your lifestyle.

12.1. The Importance of Mobility and Flexibility

Mobility and flexibility are essential components of fitness. They improve overall physical performance, decrease your likelihood of injuries, and offer a greater range of motion. However, they are often side-lined in the pursuit of strength and endurance.

Here's a brief list of exercises to boost your mobility and flexibility:

- **Hip Circles**: This aims to loosen stiff hip muscles and joints for better mobility.

- **Deep Squat Hold**: Boosts flexibility and mobility in the lower body, including the hips, glutes, and thighs.

- **Shoulder Dislocates**: Strengthens the rotator cuff and increases shoulder mobility.
- **Spinal Waves**: Aims at improving the overall mobility and flexibility of your spine.

Modify and pace these exercises as per your comfort, gradually increasing the intensity.

12.2. Fine-Tuning Your Nutrition

Fueling your body right is crucial to fortifying your fitness journey. A comprehensive guide towards this involves understanding macronutrients and micronutrients benefits. Endurance or strength-building goals will demand different metrics of macronutrients – carbs, fats, and proteins. Micronutrients help with energy production, immune function, bone health, and effectively develop and repair body tissues.

Here's a basic guide to aligning your nutrition with your fitness goals:

- **Strength Building**: High protein, moderate carbohydrates, and low fats.
- **Endurance Building**: Moderate to high carbohydrates, moderate protein, and low fats.

Remember, every body is unique and might demand a specific nutrition plan. Consider in-depth consultations with a nutritionist for personalized advice.

12.3. Crafting the Right Mindset

Ultimate fitness involves nurturing not only the body but also the mind. High-level fitness enthusiasts often employ meditation techniques to build mental resilience, concentration, and an overall balanced attitude towards life.

Meditation techniques such as mindfulness, focused meditation, and loving-kindness meditation could be beneficial starters. Practicing these regularly will promote tranquility, a positive outlook, and stress resistance, vital for any fitness enthusiast.

12.4. High-Intensity Interval Training (HIIT)

HIIT has gained prominence in recent years due to its efficient calorie-burning mechanism. It involves bursts of intense exercise followed by short, sometimes active, recovery periods. Here's a simple HIIT fitness plan:

- **Warm-up**: Do a mild, full-body warm-up for 5-10 minutes.

- **High intensity**: Choose any exercise that gets your heart rate up, such as sprinting or jumping jacks. Do it at your highest intensity for 15-30 seconds.

- **Recovery**: Rest or perform a low-intensity exercise for 45-60 seconds.

- **Repeat**: Repeat the cycle 8-10 times. Try doing HIIT workouts 2-3 times a week initially.

12.5. Advanced Practices: The Way Forward

Everything aforementioned lays the groundwork for an advanced fitness lifestyle. But it can be augmented further. Measures such as regular detailed health check-ups, keeping updated with the latest in fitness research, and trying out emerging trends like VR fitness games, cryotherapy, and air-purifying plants to enhance indoor training experiences can tip the scales in your favor.

Fostering beneficial associations will also make your fitness journey enjoyable and efficient. Surround yourself with like-minded fitness enthusiasts. Sharing knowledge and experiences with them will keep you on track and inspire new ideas.

Choosing the path of advanced fitness techniques is indeed empowering. Juggling all the elements might seem daunting initially, but rest assured, with faith, patience, and consistency, you'll see your fitness goals reaching a new zenith. So, get started, and remember - every step towards better fitness is a step towards a more adventurous life.